Reverse Diabetes

Step by step guide to reverse your diabetes today

Edith Philips

To further support this author, please post a review after you finish reading this book here https://www.amazon.com/dp/B09JBRPBG3

For all books by Edith Philips please go to
Amazon's Edith Philips page

To find out when Edith Philips has new books available and to be informed of free promotions being run by this author, please sign up for the newsletter

Edith Philips Newsletter https://bit.ly/ebk21

Other books here https://amzn.to/3yuDmVq

Free bonus.... Keto Diet and weight loss book, **download 100% free here** Also I'm given you a free copy of my weight loss book here (the best way to lose weight fast the secret to anti-aging) 100% free

Weight loss - the best way to lose weight fast, click here to download it for free https://bit.ly/3LpG3OD

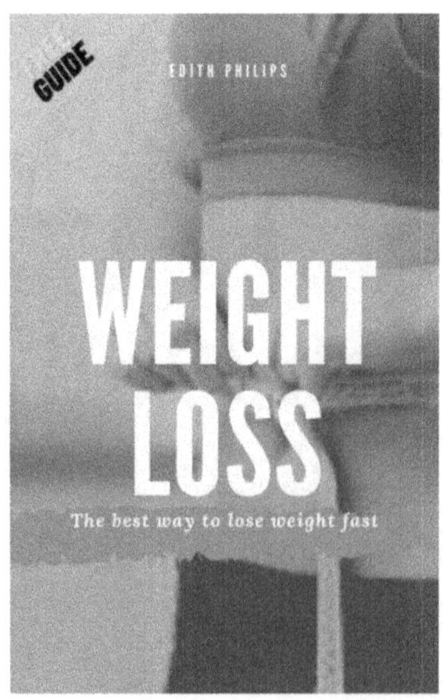

Go down below for other Free bonus offer....

Copyright © 2021

All Rights Reserved.

I want to thank you for getting this eBook, it's my pleasure. I am glad you did because I am optimistic that it will benefit you if you practice what is here.

Table of contents

Introduction

Not long ago, the American Diabetes Association (ADA) announced that reducing carbohydrate intake is the most effective nutritional strategy for improving blood sugar control in diabetic patients. Studies have shown that a low-carbohydrate diet is a safe and effective option for the treatment of type 2 diabetes. This set of evidence includes systematic reviews and meta-analysis of randomized controlled trials (according to our rating, the quality of the evidence is the highest)

A 2017 meta-analysis found that a low-carbohydrate diet reduced the need for diabetes medications and also improved certain biomarkers in patients with type 2 diabetes, including hemoglobin A1c (HbA1c), triglycerides, and blood pressure The decrease in toxic substances; and the increase in high-density lipoprotein (HDL) cholesterol (sometimes referred to as "good" cholesterol)

In addition, in a non-randomized Vita Health trial, subjects with type 2 diabetes in the intervention group followed a very low-carbohydrate diet and received remote monitoring by doctors and health coaches.

One year later, 94% of the low-carb group reduced or stopped using insulin. In addition, 25% of people have HgbA1c in the normal range without any medication, indicating that their disease is in remission, and another 35% have reached the same level when taking metformin alone.

At the two-year mark, a high proportion of subjects continued to show continuous improvement in blood glucose control. Other interventions have also shown effectiveness in inducing remission of type 2 diabetes, although there is a lack of consistency in how different trials define "remission."

The Direct trial reported that strict calorie restriction (approximately 850 calories a day) resulted in 46% relief within one year.

Bariatric surgery shows that within ten years of surgery, the remission rate of diabetes is between 25% and 50%
This evidence suggests that type 2 diabetes is not necessarily a progressive and irreversible disease. This is obviously a treatable disease.

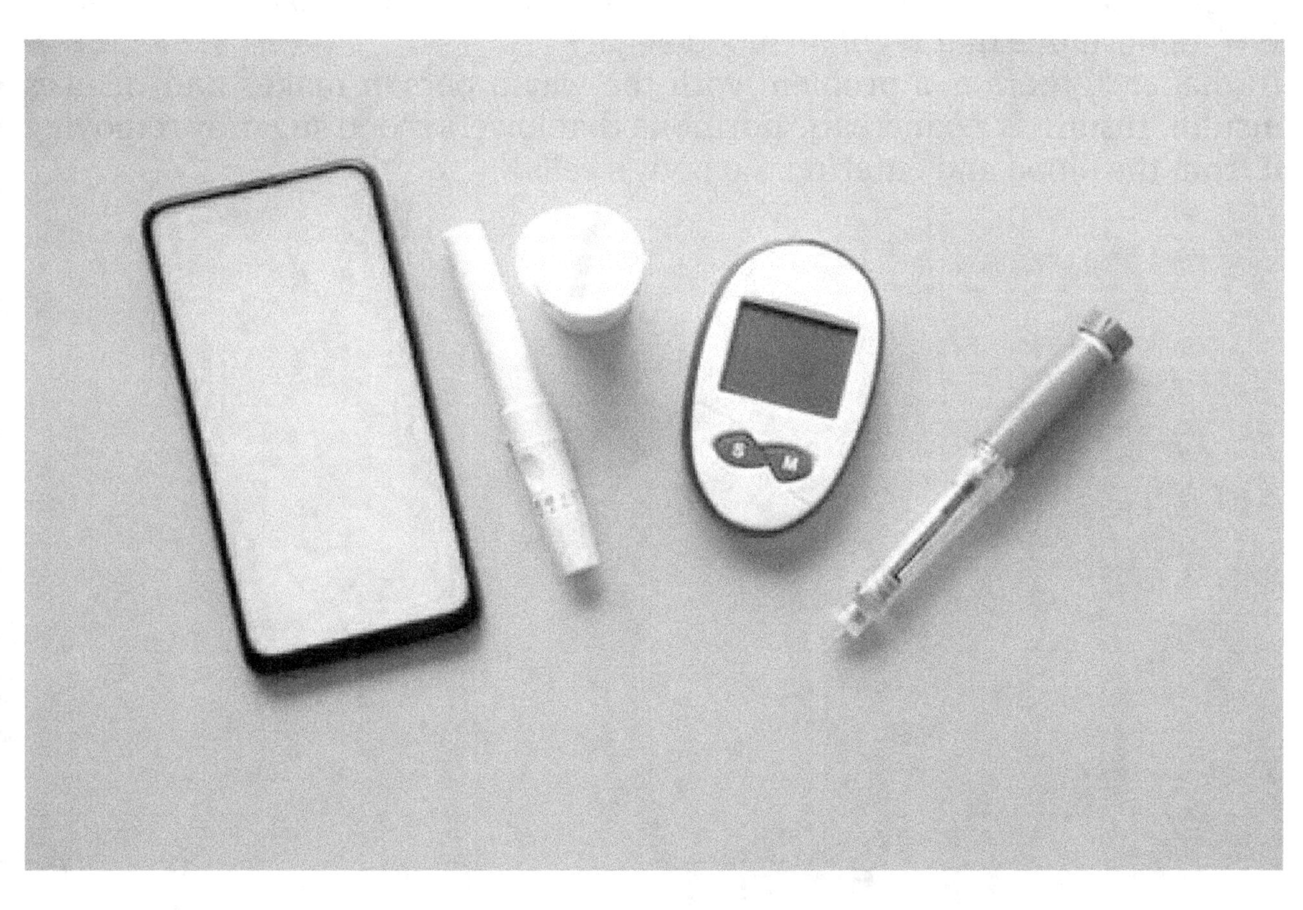

What is diabetes?

Simply put, diabetes is a blood sugar (glucose) and insulin disorder. It is a medical condition that causes high blood sugar due to a lack of insulin (a hormone that regulate blood sugar)

In diabetes, there is a problem with the way a person makes and/or uses insulin. Insulin is a pancreatic hormone that lowers blood sugar by removing it from the blood and entering the body's cells.

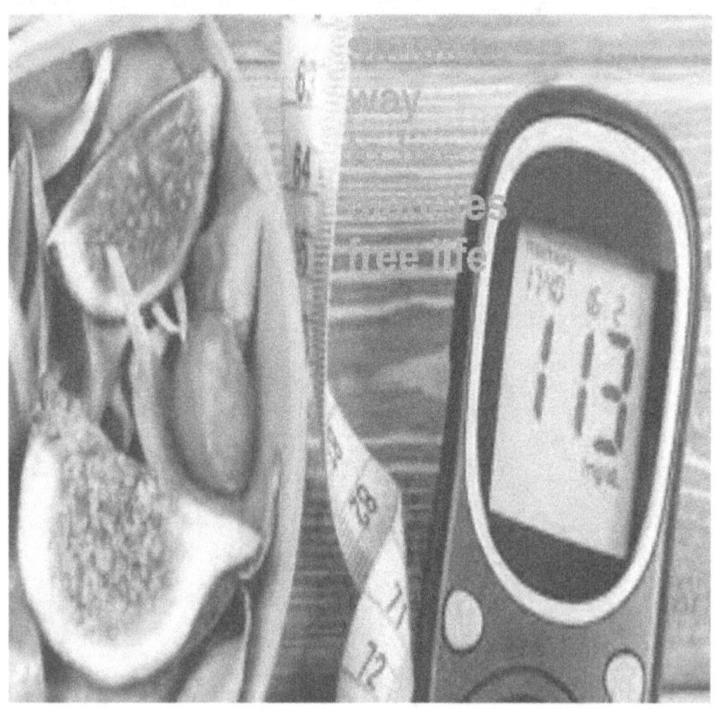

A related and very important condition is prediabetes, in which blood sugar levels are higher than normal but not high enough to be classified as diabetes. Also, insulin levels tend to rise before and after eating.

Over time, prediabetes can develop into type 2 diabetes; however, even if the blood sugar level remains within the prediabetic range, it will carry some of the same health risks as diabetes.

Although prediabetes patients generally do not have symptoms of high blood sugar, they may have some more subtle symptoms.

What is type 1 diabetes?

The body's immune system mistakenly destroys the pancreatic cells that make insulin. Because of this, patients with type 1 diabetes can no longer produce insulin on their own, and must be injected daily, not only to control blood sugar, but also to survive.

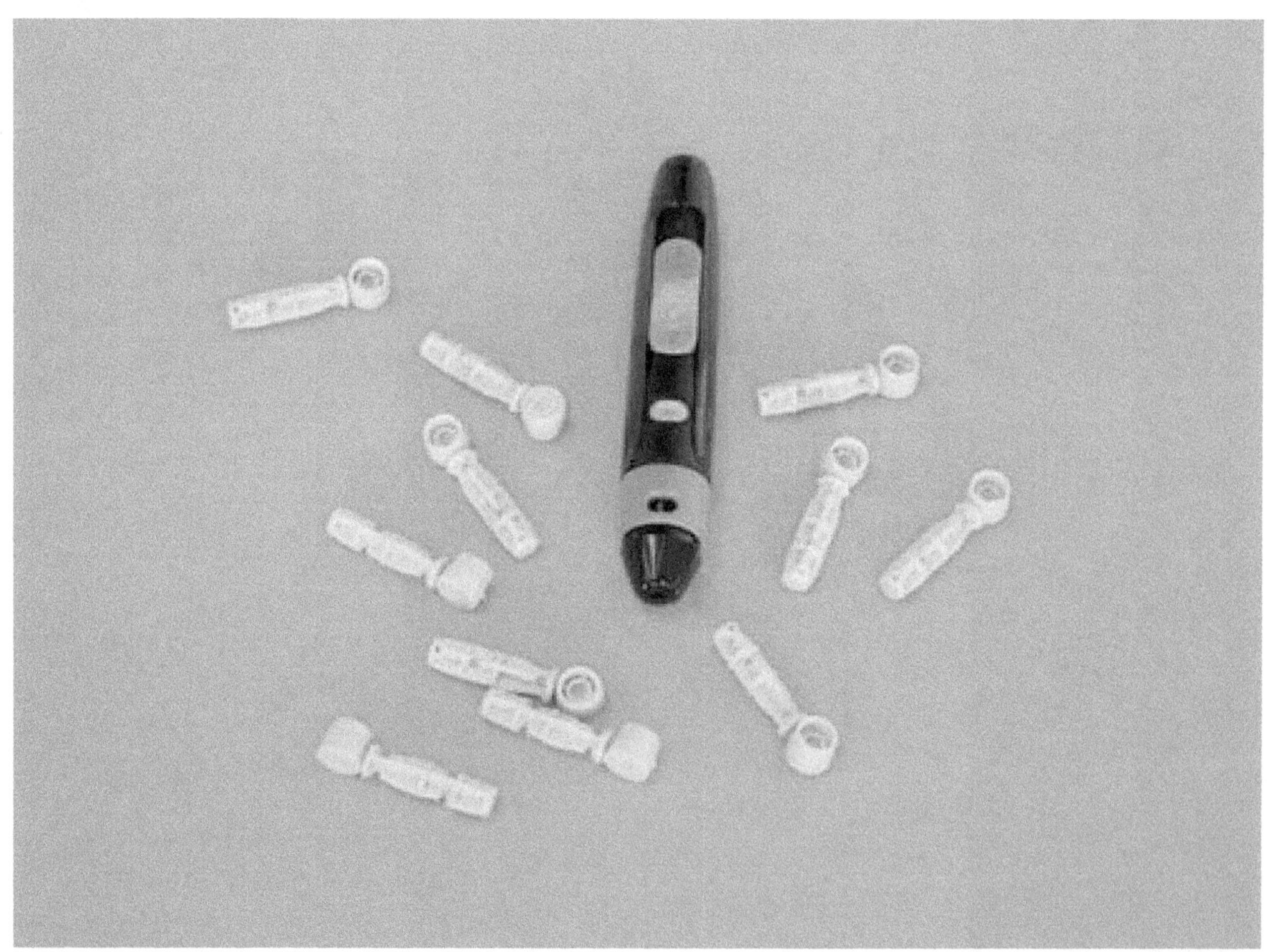

What is type 2 diabetes?

Your pancreas makes a hormone called insulin.

When your blood sugar-glucose level rises, your pancreas releases insulin. This causes the sugar to be transferred from the blood to the cells, where it can be used as an energy source. As the blood glucose level drops, the pancreas will stop releasing insulin.

Type 2 diabetes affects the way you metabolize sugar. Your pancreas cannot produce enough insulin, or your body has developed resistance to its effects. This can cause glucose to accumulate in the blood. This is called **hyperglycemia.**

When the insulin-producing cells of the pancreas are damaged, the pancreas can no longer spontaneously release enough insulin to overcome the body's resistance to it, and blood sugar levels will rise.

Symptoms of diabetes

- Erectile dysfunction
- Excessive thirst and urination
- Fatigue
- Increased hunger
- Skin rashes
- Weight loss despite eating more
- Slow healing of infection
- Urinary infections and yeast
- Blurred vision
- Skin in certain parts of the body Darker in color

You may have one, two or more symptoms, or you may not have any symptoms. The absence of symptoms does not mean that there is no diabetes.

However, understanding the common symptoms allows for an earlier diagnosis, which helps prevent long-term complications.

Is Type 2 Diabetes Reversible?

Type 2 diabetes is a serious, long-term disease. It occurs primarily in adults, but as obesity rates increase in all age groups, it becomes increasingly common in children.

There are many factors that could cause type 2 diabetes. But being overweight or obese is the biggest risk factor.

Type 2 diabetes can be life threatening. But if taken seriously, it can be controlled or even reversed.

Can you reverse type 2 diabetes?

Treatment of type 2 diabetes includes:

Control your blood sugar levels

Use medication or insulin when needed

Your doctor also recommends diet and exercise to lose weight. Some diabetes medications have weight loss-related side effects, which can also help treat or control diabetes.

To help control your diabetes, consider these:

Eat a healthy, balanced diet

Exercise

Lose excess weight

Losing weight is the main factor in reversing type 2 diabetes, because excess body fat affects insulin and how to use it.

In a small study conducted, some patients with type 2 diabetes drastically reduced their caloric intake in about 6 weeks, thus reversing their progress. The researchers pointed out that this is a small sample, and the participants only lived in this situation for a few more years.

Other research: Reliable sources indicate that bariatric surgery can reverse type 2 diabetes. This is one of the few ways to reverse diabetes in the long term. However, the methods to lose weight and reduce symptoms are not so drastic. **Exercise and diet changes may be all you need.**

Click Here https://bit.ly/3docrev to watch a video on youtube where you will learn How A 43 Yr Old US Lady Reversed her Type 2 Diabetes

Simple ways to control diabetes

Exercise
Starting exercise is important to your overall health, but it will also help you lose weight and begin to reverse your symptoms. Talk to your doctor before making a plan and remember the following:

Start slowly: If you are not used to exercising, start by walking short distances. Gradually increase the duration and intensity.

Hurry up: Slow walking is a good way to exercise. Slow walking is easy to do and does not require any equipment.

Check your blood sugar before, during and after exercise.

Take snacks with you in case your blood sugar drops during exercise.

Changing your diet
Eating a nutritious diet is another important way to help you:

Lose weight

Control your symptoms

Reverse the course of your diabetes

Your doctor can help you plan a healthy and balanced diet, or may recommend a nutritionist.

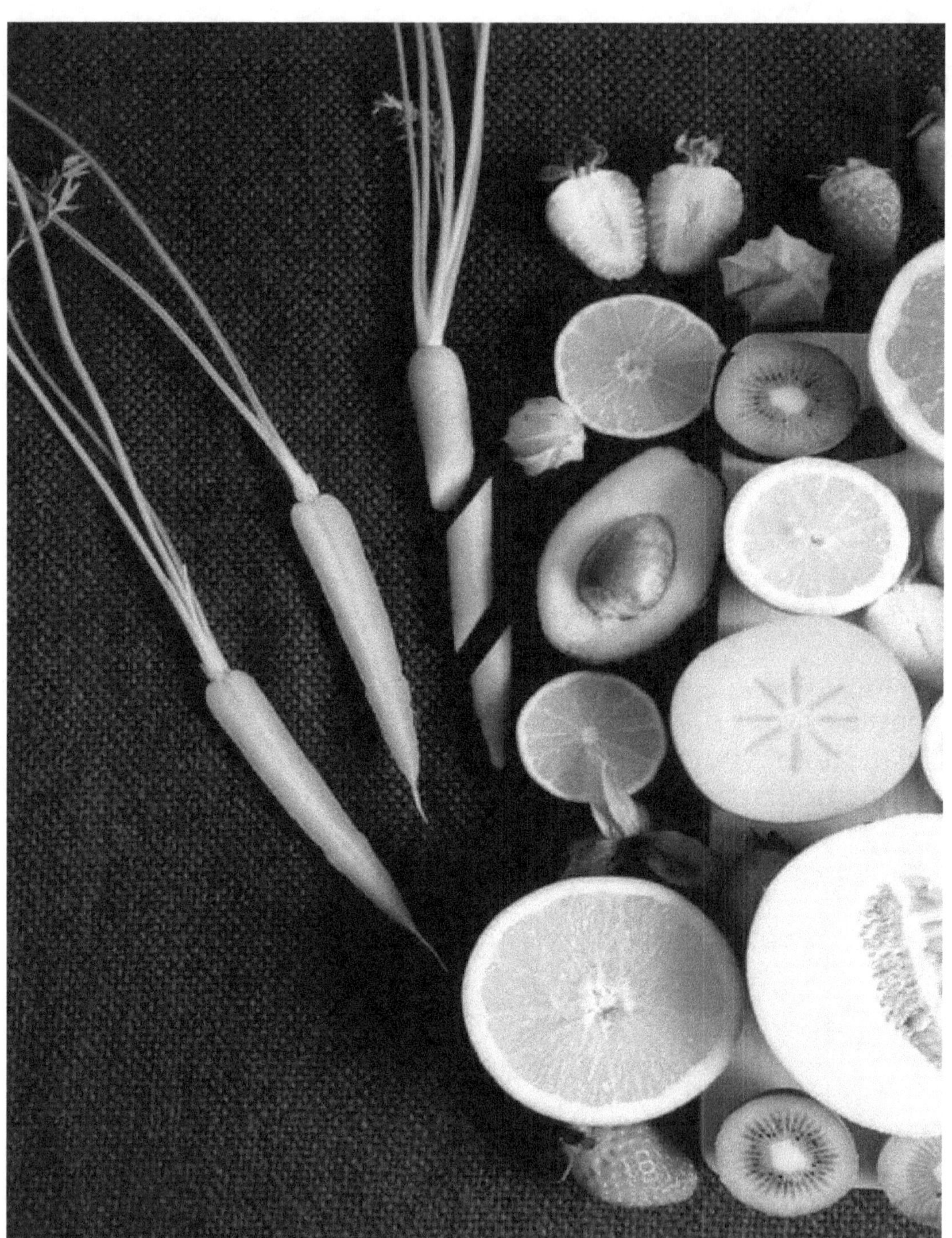

Diet to help you control or reverse diabetes

Reduce calories, especially carbohydrates
Healthy fats
Various fresh or frozen fruits and vegetables
Whole grains
Lean protein, such as poultry, fish, dairy products, low fat, Soybeans and legumes
Limit alcohol
Limit sweets

The American Diabetes Association recommends a low-carbohydrate diet, but currently does not recommend the gram standard.

However, a low-carbohydrate diet recommends that you consume the same amount of carbohydrates per meal, about 45 to 60 grams, for a total of about 200 grams per day. Eat as little as possible, which is better.

Some doctors and scientists support the ketogenic diet as a way to lose weight and stabilize blood sugar levels. The diet significantly discourages carbohydrates, usually less than 50 grams per day.

Without carbohydrates, the body is forced to break down fat for fuel. This leads to rapid weight loss and positive benefits of triglyceride and blood sugar control.

However, some diet has some negative effects, including:
Muscle cramps
Bad breath
Changes in bowel habits
Energy loss
Increased cholesterol levels
In addition, recent studies have shown that a ketogenic diet increases liver insulin resistance. And may lead to deficiencies of certain essential

micronutrients. More research is necessary on the safety and effectiveness of long-term use of this diet.

Type 2 diabetes can be reversed, but it requires a meal plan, healthy eating, and regular exercise. If you can do this and lose weight, you may be able to get rid of diabetes and its complications.

The difference between type 2 diabetes and type 1 diabetes

Type 1 diabetes is similar to type 2 diabetes, but it occurs normally in childhood and is mostly independent of weight or diet. The exact cause of type 1 diabetes is not yet clear. The most important risk factors are genetics and family history.

If you have type 1 diabetes, your pancreas produces almost no insulin. You must inject insulin regularly to metabolize glucose.

There is no cure at the moment for type 1 diabetes, and it cannot be reversed. But it can be managed. The symptoms are the same as type 2 diabetes.

If left uncontrolled or treated, both conditions can lead to serious complications, including:

Heart disease

Nerve damage

Atherosclerosis

Vision problems and blindness

Kidney damage

Skin and mouth infections

Foot infections, this can lead to amputation

Osteoporosis

Hearing problems

Whether you have type 1 or type 2 diabetes, be sure to consult your doctor before starting any new treatment and management options. Your doctor can help you develop the best plan to meet your health care needs.

How to test for blood sugar

How do you know if you have got too much sugar in your blood? If you don't know yet, you can easily perform the test in a few seconds, whether it's in your doctor's office or using your own cheap blood glucose meter.

Check your own blood glucose readings with these ranges:

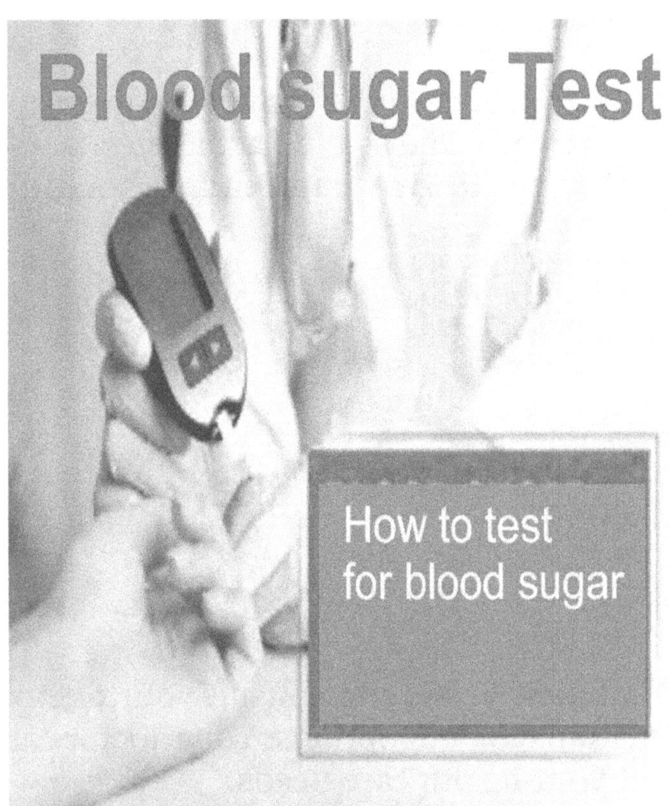

Normal blood glucose: Less than 100 mg/dL (5.6 mmol/L) after an overnight fast, and 140 mg/dL (7.8 mmol/L) after two hours of fasting Mol/L)

Pre-diabetes: 100-125 mg / dL (5.67.0 mmol / L) after an overnight fast

Diabetes: 126 mg / dL (7.0 mmol / L) or more after an overnight fast, or more than 200 mg / dL (11.1 mmol) / L) at any time
Mg = milligram
Dc = deciliter
mmol) / L = millimoles per liter

Please note that you should not use meter readings alone to diagnose diabetes or pre-diabetes. If the blood glucose meter shows that your blood sugar is high, ask your doctor to perform a blood test to confirm the diagnosis. In addition, most guidelines state that a single abnormal blood glucose reading is not enough to ensure a diagnosis of diabetes; at least two are required.

BLOOD SUGAR LEVEL CHART

	FASTING	JUST ATE	3 HOURS AFTER EATING
NORMAL	80-100	170-200	120-140
PRE-DIABETIC	101-125	190-230	140-160
DIABETIC	126+	220-300	200+

How to lower blood sugar with healthy diet

What happens if you eliminate foods that raise blood sugar from your diet? Is there something delicious to eat? We think so. Here, we have a comprehensive guide to the best foods for managing diabetes.

Many patients with type 2 diabetes now choose a diet based primarily on low carbohydrate foods, and many physicians have begun to accept it.
People with type 2 diabetes usually notice that their blood sugar levels increase from the first meal. The demand for medicines, especially insulin, is usually drastically reduced. What followed was a lot of weight loss and improvement in health indicators.

Finally, people generally feel better, more energetic and alert.
Choosing low-carbohydrate foods is an effective way to help you control blood sugar, and it is safe for most people. However, if you are taking medication for diabetes, you should work with your healthcare provider to adjust your medications when you change your diet, because the need for medications (especially insulin) can be greatly reduced.
If you are looking for a doctor who can work with you to manage diabetes by changing your diet, our guide can help you find one.

I would recommend you **Click Here** , it will take you to a video on youtube where you will learn How A 43 Yr Old US Lady Reversed Type 2 Diabetes

https://bit.ly/3docrev

https://bit.ly/3docrev

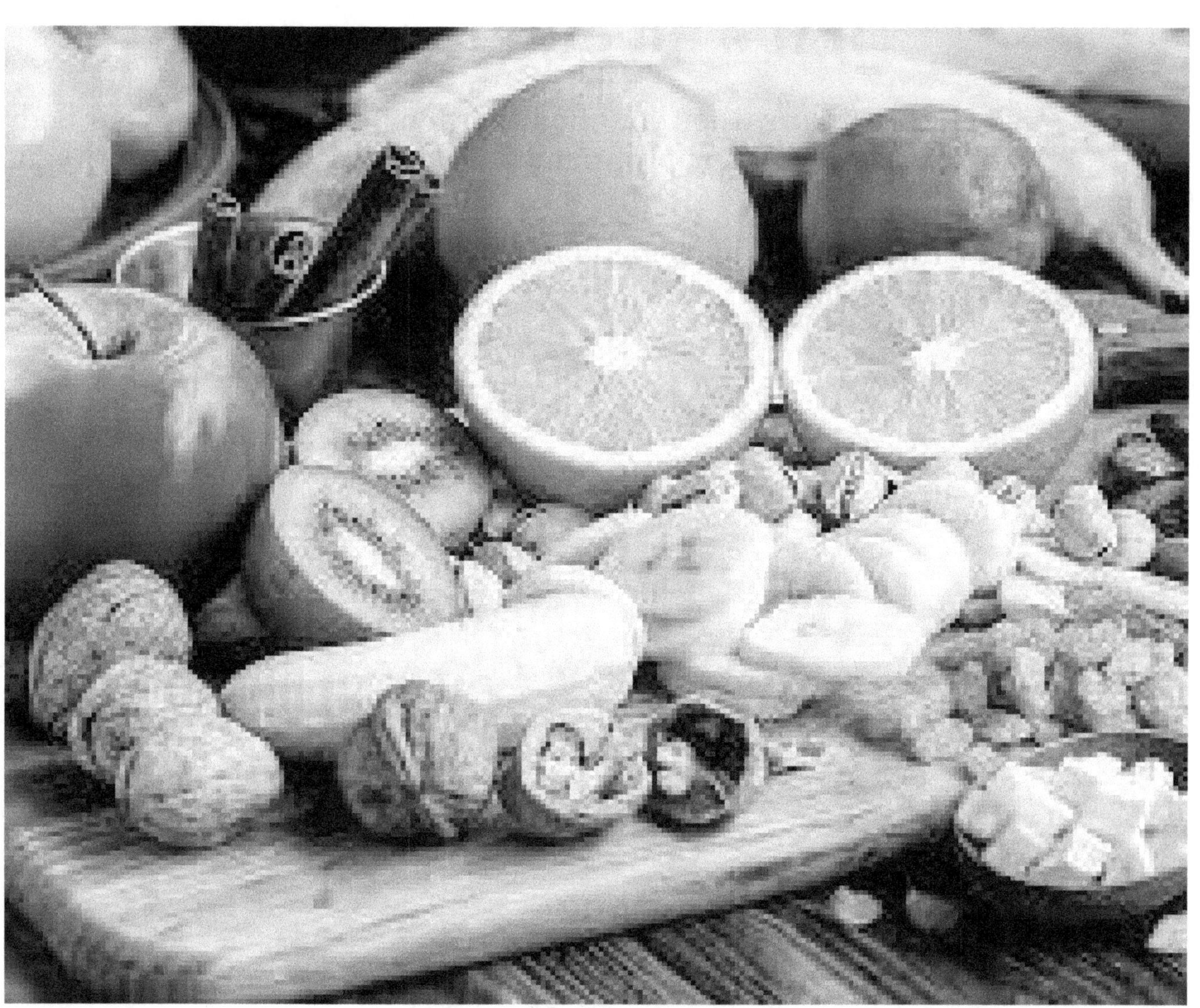

How to bring down your blood sugar if it's an emergency

High glucose occurs when your body has too little insulin, or your body can't utilize insulin appropriately. Taking insulin can bring your glucose levels down.

Drinking water is another quick method to bring down your blood sugar

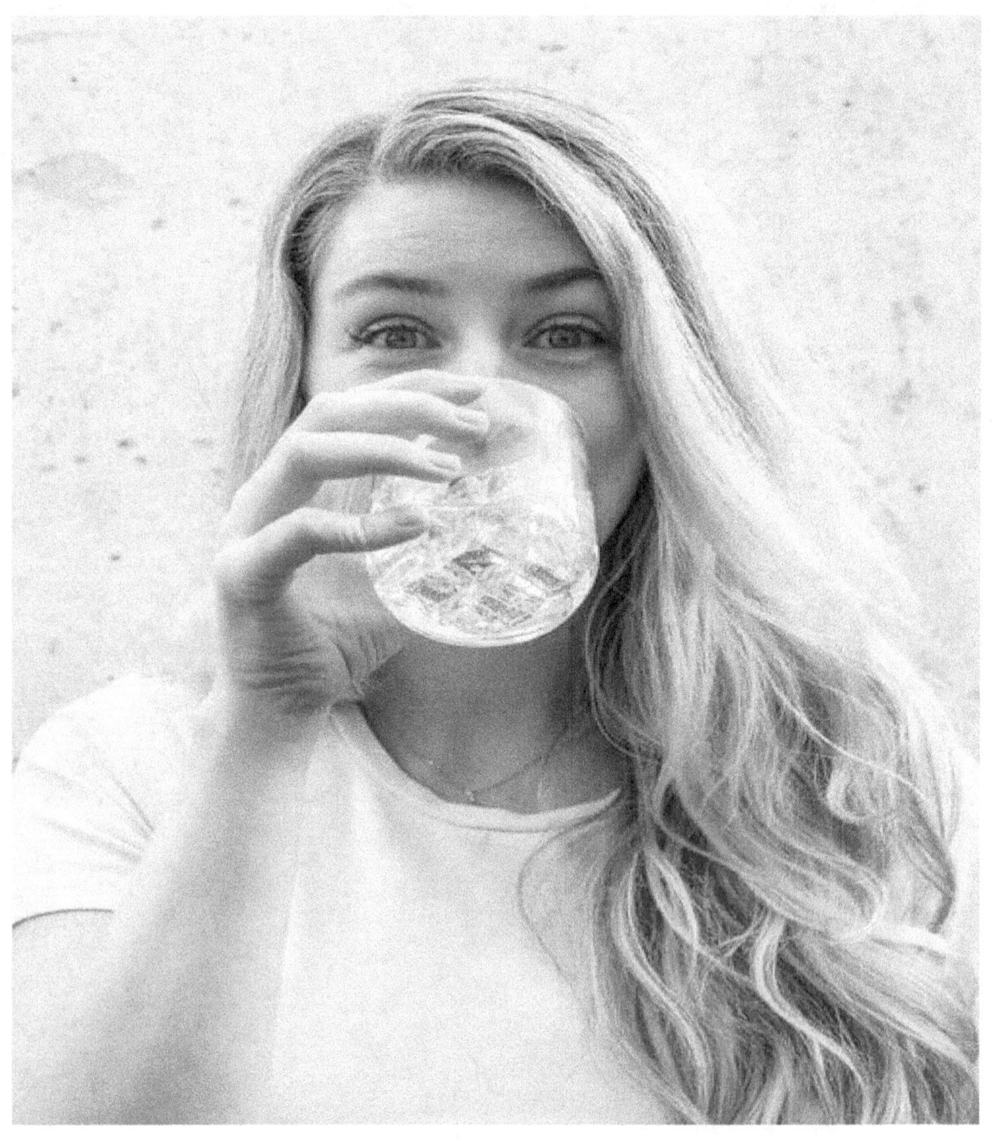

Conclusion

Just 50 years ago, type 2 diabetes was extremely rare. Now, worldwide, the number of diabetic patients is increasing rapidly and is approaching 500 million people. This is certainly a worldwide epidemic that needs attention. In the past, type 2 diabetes was considered a progressive disease with no hope of reversal or remission. People have been taught, and sometimes still, to "control" type 2 diabetes, rather than trying to reverse the underlying process.

But now type 2 diabetes patients can hope to regain health! Today we know that the characteristics of type 2 diabetes - high blood sugar and high insulin levels - can generally be reversed with a very low carbohydrate diet, strict calorie restriction, or bariatric surgery.

People don't just need to "control" the progression of diabetes. Instead, they can usually lower their blood sugar to normal through diet alone, and they can avoid or stop using most medications.

A normal blood sugar level and less or no medication may mean that the disease has not progressed and complications have not progressed. People diagnosed with type 2 diabetes can live long and healthy lives, with intact toes, eyes, and kidneys!

If you are not taking any medications, you can begin your journey to health today. If you are taking medications for diabetes or other conditions, consult your doctor before beginning any lifestyle changes (such as a low-carbohydrate diet) so that your medications will be safely adjusted as your blood sugar improves.

If you want to learn more about how to improve your health and that of your family, start here for the latest news in the following areas

Bonus tips

High glucose do occur when your body has too little insulin, or your body can't utilize insulin appropriately. Taking insulin can bring your glucose levels down.

Blood sugar comes from two places: your liver and the food you eat. You cannot control the amount of sugar made by your liver, but you can control the food you eat.

Food consists of three main categories of macronutrients (major nutrients): carbohydrates, proteins, and fats. Many foods are combinations of two or all three macronutrients, but we often group foods based on whether they are primarily carbohydrates, protein, or fat.

Again drinking water can also help to lower your blood sugar when in an emergency above all call for help or visit the clinic for physician's guidance.

Thank you for reading my book

Please post a review here https://www.amazon.com/dp/B09JBRPBG3

Edith Philips is a Bestselling Author and has written books on different titles which are available on Amazon. Click here to visit my Amazon book sales page **https://amzn.to/3yuDmVq**

To find out when Edith Philips has new books available and to be informed of free promotions being run, please sign up for newsletter

Edith Philips Newsletter https://bit.ly/ebk21

Do you want to lower your blood sugar without diet and crazy exercise and even reverse your type 2 diabetes click here to Watch these video now

Also you can get a free copy of my weight loss book here, 100% free

Keto Diet and weight loss book, **download 100% free here**

More bonus offer:

Do you want traffic to promote your content or social media offer?
Read and sign up free now, **100% Free!**

>>CLICK HERE<< to see the #1 tool that thousands of successful amazon sellers have used to make over $100,000 per month as amazon sellers, download copy 100% free.

Thank you for reading my book

Please drop a review here https://www.amazon.com/dp/B09JBRPBG3

A good friend of mine in the fitness industry told me about this diet that i had to check out and I would see result in less than two weeks. And let me tell you, this diet program truly worked. My friend is super happy, LOL

Check out this FREE video report on losing weight in two weeks at https://thoughtful-pioneer-9518.ck.page/899f3c7046. This proven system to lose weight in 2 weeks is incredible and you will be amazed with the results and say bye to that belly fat!

This proven system works and you will be amazed on how quickly you see results. Forget 4 weeks, do it in 2!

Good luck!

I'd love to hear about your results

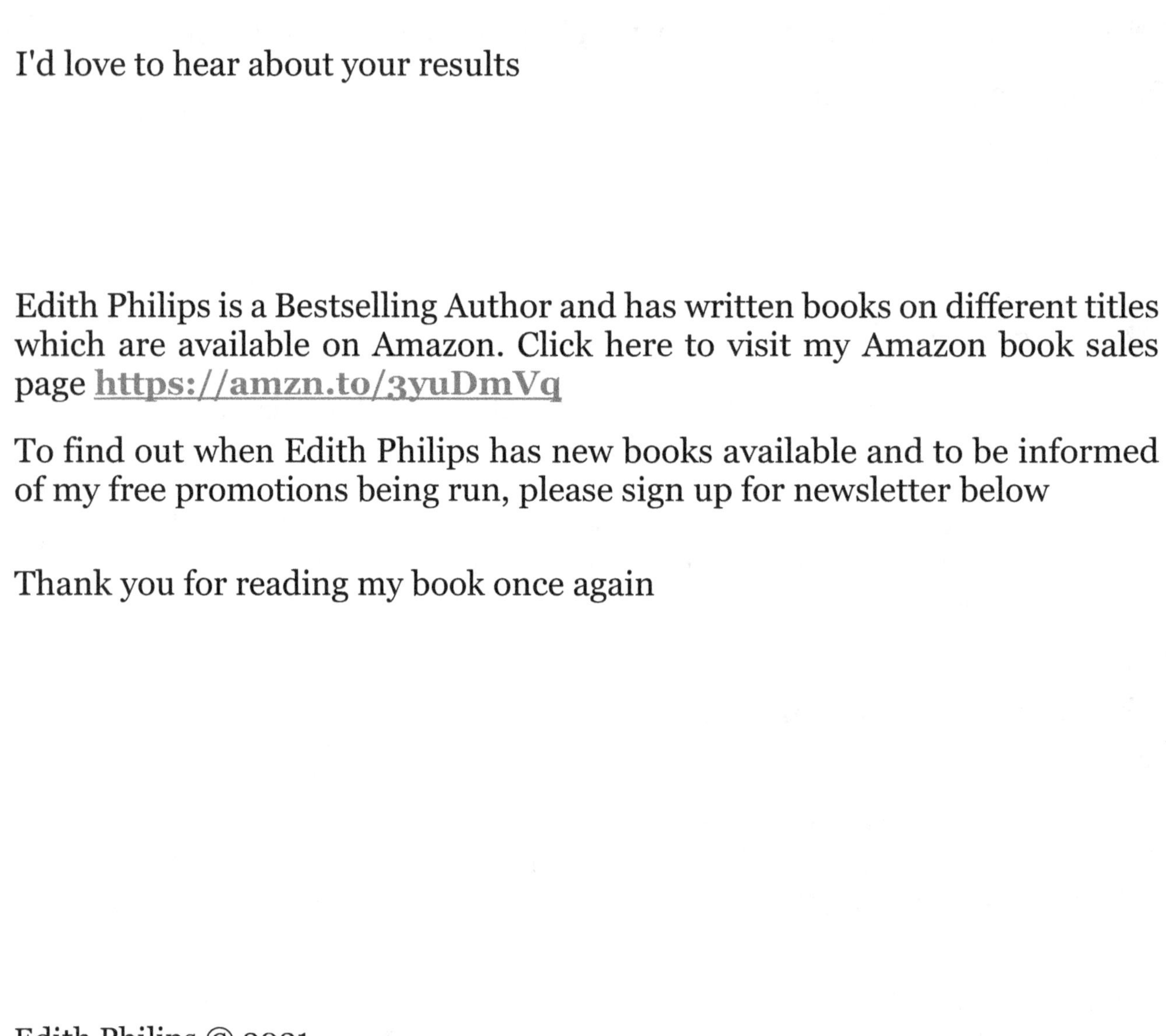

Edith Philips is a Bestselling Author and has written books on different titles which are available on Amazon. Click here to visit my Amazon book sales page https://amzn.to/3yuDmVq

To find out when Edith Philips has new books available and to be informed of my free promotions being run, please sign up for newsletter below

Thank you for reading my book once again